Mediterranean Top Recipes

A Collection of 50 Delicious Mediterranean Recipes to Enjoy Your Everyday Meals

Marta Kackson

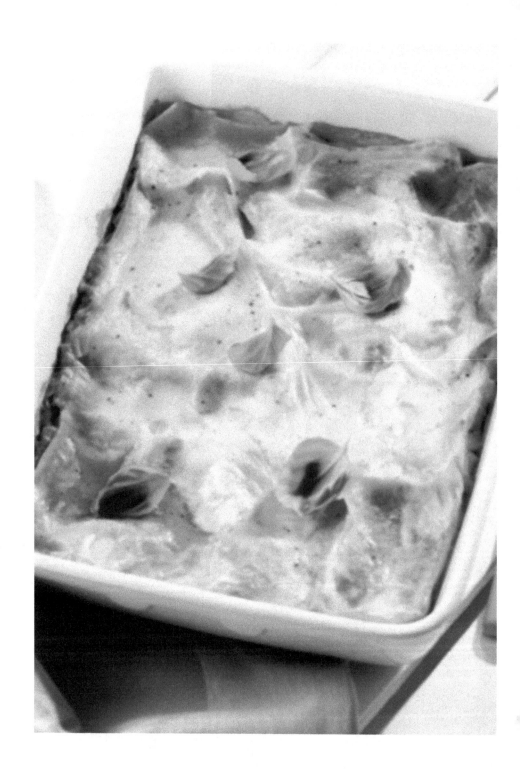

By reading this document, the reader agrees that under no circumstances is the author responsible for any losses, direct or indirect, which are incurred as a result of the use of information contained within this document, including, but not limited to, — errors, omissions, or inaccuracies.

Table of Contents

Lobster burger

Ingredients

- 2 ripe tomatoes
- 800g of cooked lobsters
- Olive oil
- 1 heaped teaspoon of Dijon mustard
- ½ a fresh red chili
- 4 thin rashers of smoked streaky bacon
- Red wine vinegar
- 4 burger buns
- 1 clove of garlic
- 1 red onion
- Tomato ketchup
- Mayonnaise
- Extra virgin olive oil
- 1 lemon
- 1 handful of watercress
- 1 soft round lettuce

Directions

- Grate the tomatoes to a slurry on both sides, discarding the seeds and skin.

- Grate in the chili, season well.
- Then, add olive oil, a swig of vinegar, and stir in bit of fresh herbs.
- Slice the lobster after twisting off the tails.
- Leave the shell on.
- Toss the chunks in olive oil, sea salt, black pepper, and mustard.
- Let barbecue for 3 minutes on each side until cooked. Peel.
- Also, barbecue the bacon, turning frequently till golden and crispy.
- Toast the buns at the same time, then lay the bottom halves on a nice board.
- Rub garlic over each side of halved buns.
- Drizzle with oil, then add a tiny blob of ketchup, with bit of mayo and a squeeze of lemon juice.
- Place the lettuce leaves, one onto each bun with a wodge of watercress.
- Top with the lobster and salsa, then, crumble over the bacon.

- Scatter over some sliced red onion, topping with the bun lid.
- Secure the burgers with skewers.
- Serve and enjoy.

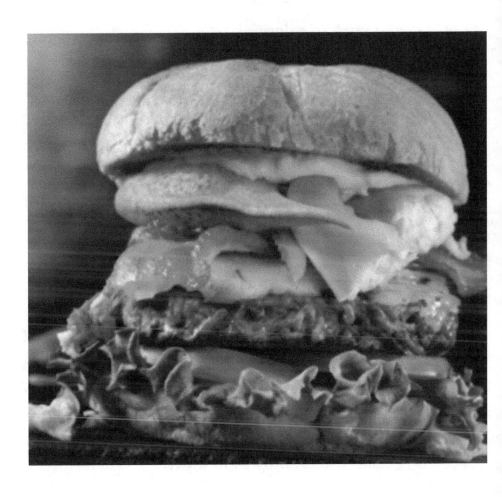

Grilled lobster rolls

Ingredients

- 2 tablespoons of mayonnaise
- 85g of butter
- 6 submarine rolls
- 1 stick of celery
- ½ of an iceberg lettuce
- 500g of cooked lobster meat

Directions

- Preheat a griddle pan until really hot.
- Butter the rolls on both sides and grill until toasted on both sides and lightly charred.
- Combine the celery, chopped lobster meat with the mayonnaise.
- Season with sea salt and black pepper to taste.
- Open warm grilled buns, shred and pile the lettuce inside each one.
- Then, top with the lobster mixture.
- Serve and enjoy right away.

Charred prawns in sweet aubergine sauce

Ingredients

- 2 aubergines
- 4 cloves of garlic
- Olive oil
- 2 large bunches of fresh basil
- 1kg of ripe tomatoes
- 1 teaspoon of dried oregano
- 2 fresh red chilies
- 3 tablespoons of red wine vinegar
- 16 king prawns

Directions

- Combine garlic, basil leaves, chilies, red wine vinegar, olive oil, and seasoning in a blender, process to a paste.
- Remove the prawn shells, then, cut along the back of each, and open up like a book.
- Place into a bowl with basil paste, mix to coat.
- Cover the bowl with Clingfilm, let marinate in the fridge for overnight.

- Score a cross in the top of each tomato, place in a large bowl and cover with boiling water.
- Drain the tomatoes, peel the skins, chop the flesh. Set aside.
- Place a saucepan over a medium heat, add olive oil.
- Add aubergines and fry for 10 minutes, stirring frequently.
- Add the remaining chili, garlic, oregano, and basil stalk into the pan, fry briefly, stir in the tomatoes.
- Add a few splashes of water, let simmer over low heat for about 30 minutes.
- Place a griddle pan over a high heat.
- Once hot enough, cook the prawns for 2 minutes on each side.
- Drop the prawns into the sauce.
- Stir the remaining basil leaves into the sauce.
- Serve and enjoy.

Spicy prawn curry with quick Pilau rice

Ingredients

- 1 teaspoon of cumin seeds
- 1 small red onion
- 1 teaspoon of unsalted butter
- ½ a bunch of fresh coriander
- 5cm piece of ginger
- 1 onion
- 1 fresh green chili
- ½ mug of basmati rice
- olive oil
- 1 teaspoon of mustard seeds
- vegetable oil
- Turmeric
- 2 ripe tomatoes
- 200g of raw king prawns, shells on
- 1 fresh bay leaf
- 100ml of light coconut milk
- 3 cardamom pods
- 4 cloves

Directions

- Heat 1 tablespoon of olive oil over a medium heat.
- Add the red onion together with the coriander stalks, and dried spices, then fry for 1 minute.
- Add the chopped ginger with the green chili, then cook for a further 5 minutes, stirring occasionally.
- Add onion with vegetable oil and butter to a pan over a medium heat.
- Let cook for 5 minutes, then, place a kettle of water on to boil.
- Sprinkle in the spices, let cook for 1 minute.
- Raise the heat, then, add the rice, stir well, add water twice the size of the rice mug, cook over reduced heat with a pinch of salt.
- Simmer for 15 minutes over a low heat, or until the water has been absorbed.
- Add the fresh tomatoes to the spiced onions with a splash of boiling water.
- Bring to the boil, season, then simmer for 5 minutes.

- Stir in the prawns together with the coconut milk, let cook for 5 minutes.
- Fluff, serve and enjoy with the curry and scattering the coriander leaves on top.

Clams casino

Ingredients

- 1 knob of unsalted butter
- 10 large cherrystone clams
- 1 lemon
- 4 large cloves of garlic
- 200g of fresh white breadcrumbs
- ½ a bunch of fresh thyme
- Extra virgin olive oil
- 4 jarred red peppers
- 8 rashers of smoked streaky bacon

Directions

- Preheat the grill to high.
- Place a deep pan over a high heat.
- Add the clams with a splash of water, cover.
- Let cook over a high heat, shaking now and then, until all the clams have opened, let cool on a tray.
- Snip each bacon rasher into 3, place the pieces in a non-stick frying pan.

- Cook over a medium heat until the bacon is just starting to crisp.
- Lift the pieces of bacon out of the pan onto a plate, return the pan to the heat.
- Add the butter together with the garlic and thyme, then add the breadcrumbs when sizzling.
- Let fry for 3 minutes, stirring.
- Season with sea salt and black pepper. Remove, let cool.
- Remove the clams from the shells, chop into quarters.
- Place into a bowl, then add a squeeze of lemon juice, a drizzle of extra virgin olive oil, and a pinch of seasoning.
- Rinse the shells, spread out on a large roasting tray.
- Place a few pepper strips into each shell, then, bit of breadcrumbs.
- Nestle a couple of clam quarters in each one and cover with more crumbs.

- Top with a piece of bacon and drizzle extra virgin olive oil.
- Place the tray on a low shelf under the hot grill for 5 minutes.
- Serve and enjoy with the remaining lemon wedges squeezed over.

Boiled prawn wontons with chili dressing

Ingredients

- 20ml of light soy sauce
- 225g of raw prawns
- 1 teaspoon of dried chili flakes
- 1 spring onion
- 40ml of vegetable oil
- 1cm piece of ginger
- 20ml of rice wine vinegar
- 1 tablespoon of Sichuan pepper
- 3 tablespoons of sea salt
- 1½ teaspoon of Shaoxing wine
- 3 tablespoons light soy sauce
- White sugar
- ½ teaspoon of sesame oil
- 24 fresh wonton wrappers

Directions

- Dry-roast the Sichuan pepper with 3 teaspoons of sea salt in a heavy.
- Once popping, remove, let cool.
- Then, grind to a powder in a pestle and mortar.

- Place chili flakes in a heatproof bowl.
- Heat olive oil in a small heavy-based frying pan until it shimmering, pour the oil over the chili to release the flavor.
- Stir, then let stand, uncovered, for 30 minutes.
- Sieve the oil over a bowl, then, mix with remaining dressing ingredients.
- Place the prawn meat, spring onion, ginger, and the remaining ingredients except for wonton, in a bowl.
- Place in the refrigerator for 30 minutes covered.
- Place a rounded teaspoon of prawn filling in the center of a wrapper.
- Dip your finger in some water and moisten the bottom edge of the wrapper, then fold it in half.
- Hold the wonton lengthways with the folded edge down.
- Fold in half lengthways, then lightly moisten one corner of the folded edge.

- Bring the two ends together with a twisting action, and seal.
- Bring a large pan of water to the boil.
- Then, drop the wontons, in batches, into the water, let cook for 2 minutes.
- Serve and enjoy with the dressing, and sprinkled with Sichuan seasoning, prepared at the beginning.

Prawn and crab wontons

Ingredients

- 200g of white crabmeat
- 30 wonton wrappers
- 1 fresh red chili
- 2 tablespoons of oyster sauce
- 200g of peeled raw tiger prawns
- Groundnut oil
- Sweet chili sauce
- ½ tablespoon of sesame oil
- Corn flour
- 1 ginger
- 1 clove of garlic
- ½ bunch of chives

Directions

- Combine ginger together with the garlic, chili, sliced chives, crabmeat, oyster sauce, sesame oil, and the prawn in a bowl. Mix to combine.
- Lay the wonton wrappers on a clean work surface, cover with a damp.
- Lightly dust a tray with corn flour.

- Spoon 1 teaspoon of the filling onto the middle of a wrapper.
- Brush the edges with a little water, then bring up over the filling, seal.
- Place on the flour-dusted tray, then repeat with the remaining ingredients.
- Pour boiling water into a saucepan over a medium-high heat.
- Bring to the boil.
- Cut out a circle of greaseproof paper so it fits snugly into a bamboo steamer, grease one side with oil, then place oil-side up into the steamer.
- Add the wontons in a single layer, then place the basket on top of the pan, steam for 8 minutes covered.
- Serve and enjoy with chili sauce.

Langoustines with lemon and pepper butter

Ingredients

- 100g of butter
- 1kg of fresh langoustines
- 2 teaspoons of coarse black pepper
- Olive oil
- 400 ml white wine
- 50g of fresh breadcrumbs
- 1 lemon
- 2 lemons

Directions

- Combine the lemon zest, butter, black pepper, and a pinch of salt, keep for later.
- Heat a grill to high.
- Combine the langoustines and wine in a pan.
- Bring to the boil, then lower the heat, let simmer for 5 minutes covered.
- Place your langoustines, belly-side down, on a chopping board, cut in half lengthways, discarding the black vein in the tail.

- Place, flesh-side up, on a baking tray, topping with the lemon butter, sprinkle over the breadcrumbs and drizzle with oil.
- Grate the zest from 1 lemon into a bowl.
- Place the lemon halves on the tray.
- Let grill for 10 minutes.
- Serve and enjoy sprinkled with zest and grilled lemon.

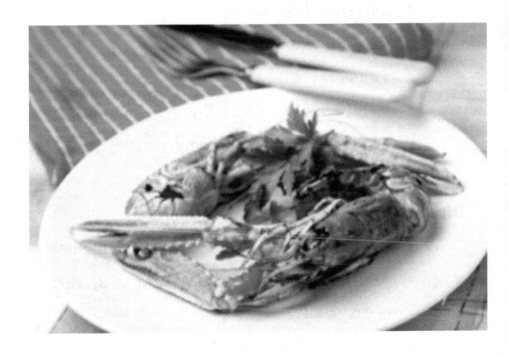

Szechuan sweet and sour prawns

Ingredients

- 150ml of unsweetened pineapple juice
- 300g of pineapple
- 1 tablespoon of low-salt soy sauce
- 1 red pepper
- 1 yellow pepper
- ½ bunch of fresh coriander
- 3 tablespoons of rice vinegar
- 2 cloves of garlic
- 2 fresh red chilies
- Sea salt
- 1 ginger
- ½ tablespoon of corn flour
- 24 peeled raw king prawns
- Groundnut oil

Directions

- Preheat a large griddle pan over a high heat.
- Add the pineapple for 4 minutes, turning occasionally.
- Remove, let cool on a board.

- Add sliced peppers to the griddle for about 3 minutes, turning halfway.
- Bash the garlic together with the chilies, and a pinch of salt to a rough paste, in a pestle and mortar.
- Add the ginger, then bash until broken down, combined.
- Place the chili paste into a large bowl with the prawns and a splash of oil, mix.
- Heat a lug of oil in a large non-stick frying pan over a medium-high heat.
- Add the prawn mixture, let fry for 4 minutes.
- Then, chop the cooled pineapple into bite-sized chunks.
- In a bowl, combine the pineapple juice together with the vinegar, soy, corn flour, and a splash of water, add to the pan along with the chargrilled pineapple and peppers.
- Bring to the boil, then, simmer over a low heat for about 2 minutes
- Serve and enjoy with steamed rice.

Cooked oyster with burnt butter

Ingredients

- ½ of a lemon
- 800g of rock salt
- 40g of unsalted butter
- 8 rock oysters
- Tabasco sauce

Directions

- Preheat the oven to the maximum heat.
- Place the rock salt into an ovenproof frying pan.
- Place the rock salt in the oven to preheat for around 20 minutes.
- Then, place in the oysters on top, return the pan to the oven for 10 minutes.
- Melt the butter in a frying pan over a medium heat, then cook for 3 minutes, or until the oyster turns to deep golden.
- Add a few drops of Tabasco to taste.
- Remove from heat, add a squeeze of lemon juice, swirling the pan until combined.

- Put the pan to one side.
- Insert an oyster knife in, then carefully lever it open.
- Discard the oyster tops, then place the bottom shells with the oyster on a platter.
- Serve and enjoy with a drizzle over the burnt butter.

Cajun blackened fish steaks

Ingredients

- 2 level teaspoons of smoked paprika
- 4 x 200g of white fish fillets
- 1 teaspoon of cayenne pepper
- Lemon
- 10 sprigs of fresh thyme
- 2 tablespoons of olive oil
- 4 sprigs of fresh oregano
- 2 cloves of garlic

Directions

- Bash the fresh herbs together with the garlic in a pestle and mortar until coarse paste forms.
- Then, mix in the spices with bit of sea salt, black pepper, olive oil, and a squeeze of the juice of half the lemon, stir well.
- Lightly score the skin of your fish in lines about 2cm apart.
- Smear the rub all over both sides of the fish.
- Place a pan over a medium-high heat.

- Place the fish in the pan, skin side down, let cook for 4 minutes.
- It will get quite smoky, so you might want to open a window.
- Lower the heat, then, flip your fish over, and continue to cook for 4 minutes on the other side.
- Cut the remaining lemon half and the second lemon into wedges.
- Serve and enjoy the fish with salad and boiled potatoes dressed in good olive oil.

Barbecued langoustines with aioli

Ingredients

- 12 langoustines
- ½ clove garlic
- 1 teaspoon of sea salt
- Lemon juice
- 1 large egg yolk
- Sprigs fennel tops
- 1 teaspoon of Dijon mustard
- 300ml of extra virgin olive oil
- Freshly ground black pepper

Directions

- To make the aioli, smash the garlic together with salt in a pestle and mortar.
- Whisk the egg yolk with the mustard in a bowl, then adding olive oils to it bit by bit, the rest.
- Add the smashed garlic with lemon juice, salt and pepper.
- Lay the langoustines flat on a chopping board, with a sharp knife, saw through their shells lengthways.

- Open them out in a butterfly style and flatten them down gently.
- Season, then cook, cut-side down, across the bars on a hot Barbie for 2 minutes, then briefly on the other side.
- Sprinkle with torn fennel tops.
- Serve and enjoy with lemony aioli.

Creamy Cornish mussels

Ingredients

- 250ml of Cornish cider
- 600g of mussels
- 1 bunch of fresh chives
- 4 cloves of garlic
- 50g of clotted cream

Directions

- Discard open mussels.
- Place a large deep pan on a high heat.
- Then, pour in 1 tablespoon of olive oil, add garlic with chives, and cider.
- Bring to a fast boil, add the mussels with the clotted cream, cover and leave for 4 minutes, shaking occasionally.
- When all the mussels have opened, they are done. Discard any closed ones.
- Taste the sauce, and adjust the seasoning with sea salt and black pepper.
- Sprinkle over the remaining chives.
- Serve and enjoy.

Pesto mussels and toast

Ingredients

- 50ml of white wine
- 70g of pesto
- 160g of fresh or frozen peas
- 2 thick slices of whole meal bread
- 500g of mussels
- 200g of baby courgettes
- 200g of ripe mixed-color cherry tomatoes
- 2 sprigs of fresh basil

Directions

- Put a large pan on a medium-high heat.
- Toast the bread as the pan heats up, turn when golden.
- Remove the toast, spread one quarter of the pesto on each slice.
- Turn on the heat under the pan to full heat.
- Place in the mussels.
- Stir in the remaining pesto, together with the courgettes, tomatoes, and peas.

- Add the wine let cover and steam for 4 minutes, shaking the pan occasionally.
- When all the mussels have opened and are soft, they are done.
- Divide the mussels, vegetables, and juices between 2 large bowls.
- Pick over the basil leaves and serve with the pesto toasts on the side.
- Enjoy.

Mussels with Guinness

Ingredients

- 1 fresh bay leaf
- ½ a bunch of fresh thyme
- 1 shallot
- 250ml of Guinness
- 2 cloves of garlic
- 2 rashers of smoked bacon
- 1kg of mussels
- 50ml of double cream
- ½ a bunch of fresh flat-leaf parsley
- 1 knob of unsalted butter

Directions

- In a pan, melt the butter and sweat the shallot with the garlic and bacon for 5 minutes.
- Add half of the herbs, together with the bay and a pinch of sea salt and black pepper.
- Then, add the mussels, then the Guinness.
- Let boil, then lower the heat, let steam for 5 minutes covered.
- Stir in the cream and remaining herbs.

- Taste, and adjust the seasoning.
- Serve and enjoy with bread.

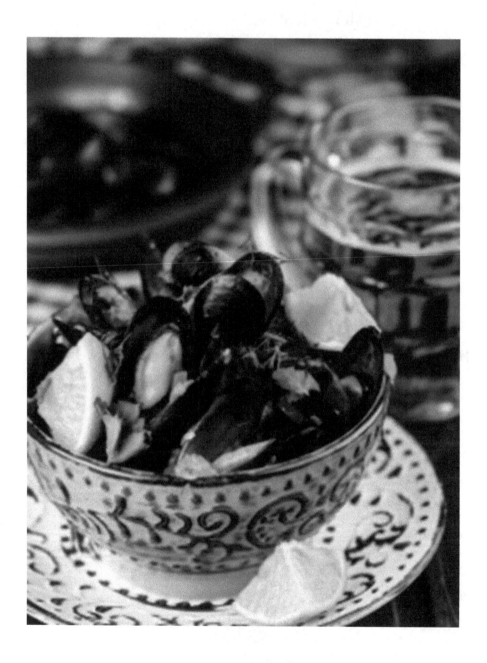

Shellfish and cider stew

Ingredients

- 1 tablespoon of unsalted butter
- 4 ripe plum tomatoes
- 3 leeks
- 600g of clams
- 600g of mussels
- 3 shallots
- 6 razor clams
- ½ a bunch of fresh flat-leaf parsley
- 500ml of organic fish stock
- 750ml of cider
- 1 teaspoon of tomato purée
- 6 langoustines
- 3 tablespoons of double cream

Directions

- Start by melting the butter in a large pan over a low heat.
- Gently fry the leeks together with the shallots, tomatoes, and parsley until soft.
- Season, then add the stock with cider.

- Raise the heat, let the liquid boil for 10 minutes, until reduces slightly.
- Warm a large serving bowl.
- Add the langoustines, cover for 3 minutes.
- Then add the razor clams. Cook for a further 2 minutes while covered.
- Add the mussels together with the clams.
- Stir gently, then, add another splash of cider, cover, let cook for a further 5 minutes, or until the mussels and clams have opened.
- Transfer the shellfish to the warmed serving bowl and put the sauce back on the heat.
- Add the cream together with the tomato purée, stir well to combine.
- Pour the sauce over the shellfish in the bowl.
- Serve and enjoy with crusty bread.

Simple baked cod with tomatoes

Simple baked cod is flavorful due to the garlic, lemon, and herbs used typically basil. It is a perfect Mediterranean Sea diet for dinner or lunch.

Ingredients

- salt, pepper and chili flakes to taste
- 3 tablespoons of olive oil
- ¼ cup of basil leaves torn
- 2 cups of cherry
- 3 garlic cloves rough chopped
- 2 lb. of cod fillets
- 1 lemon – zest and slices

Directions

- Begin by preheating your oven ready to 400°F.
- Pour the olive oil in a baking dish .
- Scatter the garlic cloves.
- Add the tomatoes with lemon slices, toss and pus to one side.
- Pat dry the fish, place in the baking dish , turn to coat each side with oil.

- Spread out the tomato garlic mixture and nestle in the fish.
- Make sure tomatoes on the sides, lemons underneath.
- Season all with <u>salt</u> , pepper and chili flakes.
- Let bake for 10 minutes, scatter with lemon zest.
- Continue to bake for 5 more minutes.
- Add the torn basil leaves, tossing with the warm tomatoes.
- Garnish every piece of fish with a wilted basil leaf.
- Serve and enjoy immediately.

Roasted salmon with braised lentils

Ingredients

- 7 garlic cloves, finely minced
- 1 tablespoon of fresh thyme
- 2 teaspoons of whole-grain mustard
- 2 cups of French Green Lentils
- Fresh thyme sprigs for garnish
- 2 teaspoons of lemon zest
- 2 bay leaves
- 5 sprigs of fresh thyme
- ¼ cup of sherry wine
- 3 teaspoon of salt
- pepper to taste
- 2 lbs. of salmon
- 1 onion, diced
- 1 cup of diced celery
- 5 tablespoon of olive oil
- 1 cup of diced carrot
- 4 cups of veggie

Directions

- Preheat heat oven to 325F.

- Pat dry the salmon.
- Combine garlic with thyme, whole grain, lemon zest, olive oil, salt and pepper in a small bowl.
- Brush a little marinade on the bottom sides of salmon.
- Then, place on parchment -lined sheet pan .
- Spoon the remaining over top, to form a thin layer. Set aside.
- Bake salmon in the preheated oven for 15 minutes or so.
- Heat oil in a large sauté pan over medium heat.
- Add onion together with the celery and carrots.
- Stir for 5 minutes, lower the heat, continue to cook for more 5 more minutes.
- Add the garlic and lentils.
- Cook for 2 minutes while stirring.
- Add the wine. Let this cook-off, about 2 minutes.
- Pour in the stock, salt , and mustard, and stir until combined, let simmer.

- Add the bay leaves and thyme sprigs, cover and gently simmer on low heat for 30 minutes.
- Taste and adjust accordingly.
- Serve and enjoy.

Moroccan salmon

The Moroccan salmon derives its flavor and taste from variety of fruits and vegetables and herbs. Mint and oranges are key healthy ingredients that elevate this Mediterranean Sea diet recipe.

Ingredients

- pinch of cayenne
- 2 salmon filets
- ½ teaspoon of cinnamon
- Orange zest
- ½ teaspoon of salt
- ¾ teaspoon of sugar
- 1 tablespoon of oil for searing
- ½ teaspoon of cumin

Directions

- Preheat oven to 350°F.
- In a small bowl, combine cinnamon together with the cumin, salt, sugar and cayenne.
- Sprinkle over both sides of the salmon.
- Heat oil in an oven proof skillet over medium temperature.

- Sear salmon on both sides for 2 minutes each side.
- Place in the warm oven to finish for 5 minutes.
- Garnish with orange zest.
- Serve and enjoy with Moroccan quinoa.

Pan seared salmon with chia seeds, fennel slaw and pickled onions

Ingredients

- ½ ounce of package dill
- ½ teaspoon of salt
- 3 tablespoon of lemon juice
- ¼ cup of thinly sliced sweet onion
- ½ teaspoon of dried mint, dill or tarragon
- ½ teaspoon of granulated garlic
- 1 Turkish cucumber
- 2 teaspoons of chia seeds
- Salt and pepper to taste
- 3 tablespoon of olive oil
- ½ lemon
- 2 6 ounces of wild Salmon
- 1 extra-large fennel bulb, thinly sliced

Directions

- Place fennel bulb, cucumber, dill, olive oil, lemon juice, lemon juice, salt and pepper in a medium bowl, toss well. Set aside.
- Brush the tops of salmon with olive oil .

- Place salt together with the pepper, dried herbs, granulated garlic, chia seeds in a small bowl, mix.
- Coat the top of the fish liberally with the chia mixture, pressing it down with fingers.
- Then, heat olive oil in a pan over medium heat.
- Let the pan get hot enough, then add the fish with chia seed side down and pan sear for 4 minutes until golden.
- Turnover, to keep crust intact and continue cooking until fish is cooked in 4 minutes.
- Serve and enjoy with a squeeze of lemon juice on top.

Ceviche

Ceviche is quite a delicious fish recipe that features cucumber, tomatoes, chilies, cilantro, lime and even avocado. As a result, the variety of vegetables makes this recipe a perfect Mediterranean Sea diet choice for any meal.

Ingredients

- 1 cup of diced cucumber
- ½ of a red onion, thinly sliced
- 1 pound of fresh fish- sea bass
- 1 fresh serrano chili pepper seeded
- 1 cup of grape
- 1 semi-firm avocado, diced
- 3 garlic cloves finely minced¼ teaspoon of black pepper
- ½ cup of fresh cilantro chopped
- 1 ½ teaspoon of kosher salt
- ¾ cup of fresh lime juice
- 1 tablespoon of olive oil

Directions

- Place fish together with the onion, garlic, salt , fresh chilies, pepper, and lime juice in a shallow serving bowl , mix.
- Transfer to a refrigerator to marinate for at 45 minutes.
- Gently toss in the fresh cilantro with cucumber and tomato.
- Drizzle with olive oil , mix.
- Taste, and adjust accordingly.
- Gently fold in the avocado at the end, after mixing everything.
- Serve and enjoy.

Seared Hawaiian ono with honey soy glaze and pineapple salsa

Ingredients

- 1 teaspoon of finely minced or grated ginger root
- 1 mild red chili
- 2 lbs. of Fresh Ono cut into 6 pieces
- ⅓ cup of soy sauce
- ⅓ cup of honey
- 3 teaspoon of sliced ginger
- ⅛ teaspoon of kosher salt
- 2 garlic cloves
- ¼ cup of finely diced red onion
- 1 teaspoon of olive oil
- zest and juice of one small lime
- ½ cup of chopped cilantro
- Pineapple Ginger Salsa
- ½ pineapple, pealed cored, small diced
- 1 jalapeño- seeds removed, diced

Directions

- Blend soy sauce together with the honey , garlic, sliced ginger, and olive oil in a blender until smooth.
- Put the fish and marinade in a Ziploc bag for 20 minutes or longer.
- Cut pineapple in half, saving top half for another use.
- Slice and dice into ½ inch cubes, then place in a medium bowl.
- Toss in the jalapeno, red chili, red onion, ginger root, cilantro, zest and juice and kosher salt.
- Taste, and adjust accordingly.
- Heat oil in a large heavy bottom skillet, over medium temperature.
- When oil is hot enough, place in the fish, saving the marinade.
- Sear the fish, on its sides, set aside.
- Pour the remaining marinade into the skillet let boil briefly.
- Strain and place in a small bowl.

- Spoon over the fish, with a generous amount of pineapple salsa.
- Serve and enjoy.

Sea bass with cannellini bean stew

A combination of beans and fish is an incredible protein blast. In 30 minutes, this Mediterranean Sea diet recipe will be just ready waiting for your bite.

Ingredients

- ½ teaspoon of kosher salt
- 2 tablespoons of olive oil
- ¼ teaspoon of cracked pepper
- 1 medium onion, diced
- Oil, salt and pepper for fish
- 1 cup of peeled, diced carrot
- 4 cups of chicken stock
- 1 cup of diced celery
- Italian parsley for garnish
- 4 smashed and roughly chopped garlic cloves
- 2 cups of diced tomatoes
- 4 four-ounce of sea bass fillets
- 3 cups of cannellini beans
- 1 cup of water
- 2 tablespoons of fresh sage

Directions

- In a medium heavy-bottomed pot, heat oil over medium heat.
- Add onions, stir for 2 minutes.
- Add carrots together with the celery and garlic, sauté over medium heat for 5 minutes, stirring occasionally.
- Add canned beans with the 2 cups of stock, herbs, tomatoes, salt and pepper, let boil.
- Lower the heat, cover, let simmer for 15 minutes.
- Heat 2 tablespoons of olive oil in a skillet, over medium temperature.
- Pat dry fish with paper towels.
- Season generously with kosher salt and pepper.
- Sear each side until a golden crust forms on the fish.
- Lower the heat, let cook through.
- Place the stew in a wide shallow dish topping with seared fish

- Serve and enjoy garnished with fresh Italian parsley.

Crispy Moroccan carrots

Ingredients

- 6 tablespoons of natural yoghurt
- 12 baby carrots
- Runny honey
- 3 oranges
- 2 teaspoons of rose harissa
- 1 tablespoon of tahini
- 3 fresh bay leaves
- 2 tablespoons of sesame seeds
- 3 sprigs of fresh thyme
- 4 sheets of filo pastry
- Olive oil

Directions

- Preheat the oven ready to 400°F.
- Place and cook the carrots in a pan of fast-boiling salted water for 10 minutes.
- Drain any excess water.
- Grate half the orange zest into the empty pan with all the juice.
- Place on a medium heat.

- Add the bay with thyme and a pinch of sea salt, let cook until syrupy.
- Fold carrots back into the glaze to coat. Let cool.
- Lay out the filo sheets rubbed with oil, then cut lengthways into 3 strips.
- Place a carrot at the bottom of each and roll up.
- Repeat for all the carrots and filo.
- Transfer to a baking tray.
- Brush each lightly with oil, let roast for 20 minutes.
- Drizzle with a little honey and scattering with the sesame seeds for last 5 minutes.
- Stack the carrots on a board, swirl the tahini and harissa through the yoghurt.
- Serve and enjoy.

Rogan josh scotch eggs

Ingredients

- mango chutney
- 5 large free-range eggs
- 2 liters of vegetable oil
- 2 x 250 g packets of mixed cooked grains
- 50g of plain flour
- 2 heaped teaspoons of Rogan josh curry paste
- 1 bunch of fresh mint
- 1 naan bread

Directions

- Start by soft-boiling 4 eggs in a pan of boiling salted water on a medium heat for 5 minutes.
- Drain, let cool under running water. Peel.
- Place the grains into a food processor with the curry paste, mint leaves, process until tacky in texture.
- Divide into 4 balls.
- Pat one at a time on a greaseproof paper.

- Place the paper flat on your hand, put a peeled egg in the center and mold the mixture up and around the egg to seal it inside.
- Remove the ball from the paper, press in hands to create the perfect covering.
- Place the flour in one bowl, beat the remaining egg in a separate bowl, add the naan to fine crumbs into a third bowl.
- Cover the coated eggs with flour, dip into the beaten egg and roll in the crumbs.
- Place on a medium-high heat.
- Lower the Scotch eggs into the pan let cook for 8 minutes.
- Scoop out and drain on kitchen paper.
- Serve and enjoy.

Moroccan salad with blood oranges, olives, almond and mint

Ingredients

- 1 teaspoon of honey , maple
- 1 ¾ cups of water
- Pinch of salt
- 12 fresh mint leaves, torn
- 2 green onions, sliced diagonally
- 1 tablespoon of red wine vinegar
- 1 cup of rinsed quinoa
- ¼ cup of thinly sliced Kalamata olives
- cracked pepper and salt to taste
- ¼ cup of toasted slivered
- 3 blood oranges- divided
- ¼ cup of olive oil

Directions

- Boil quinoa in salted water in a medium pot on the stove.
- Lower heat once boiling, cover and cook for15 minutes.

- In a medium bowl, add sliced green onions with sliced olives, and 2 oranges.

- Toss the quinoa in the bowl with the oranges.

- Dress with 4 tablespoons of olive oil , zest and juice of the remaining orange, and honey . Stir.

- Taste and adjust accordingly.

- Scatter with toasted slivered almonds and fresh torn mint leaves.

- Serve and enjoy warm or chilled.

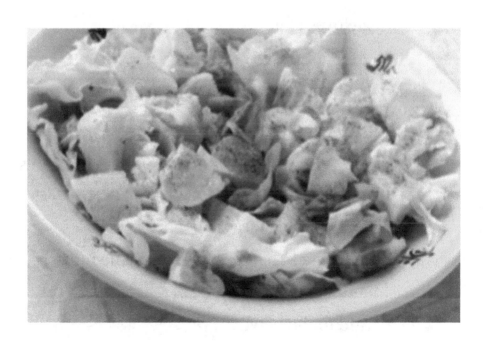

Warm grape and radicchio salad

The warm grape and radicchio salad recipe is carefully charred under the grill with incredible fresh balsamic and honey for a sweeter taste.

Ingredients

- 30g of rocket
- 200g of seedless red grapes
- 1 radicchio or 2 red chicory
- 1 tablespoon of runny honey
- 2 tablespoons of balsamic vinegar
- Olive oil
- 2 cloves of garlic
- 2 sprigs of fresh rosemary
- 2 heaped tablespoons of pine nuts

Directions

- Place grapes on a griddle pan over a high heat let grill for 5 minutes.
- Transfer in a large salad bowl.
- Working in batches, grill, char the radicchio to soften on both sides.
- Add to the bowl.

- Add garlic, rosemary leaves, pine nuts, and oil in the still-hot griddle pan.
- Add the balsamic vinegar together with the honey. Toss.
- Seasoning with sea salt and black pepper.
- Let settle for 10 minutes, then toss.
- Serve and enjoy.

Nordic nicoise salad

Ingredients

- 2 teaspoons of fresh grated
- 1 tablespoon of chopped fresh dill
- 2 eggs
- 1 cup of snap peas
- 1 cucumber
- Pinch sugar
- 1 tablespoon of finely chopped shallot
- 4 radishes
- 6 ounces of smoked trout
- 1 tablespoon of capers
- 2 tablespoons of fresh dill
- ¼ cup of olive oil
- 2 tablespoons of champagne vinegar
- 8 baby potatoes
- 1 teaspoon of wholegrain mustard
- 1 bunch watercress
- ¼ teaspoon of salt
- ¼ teaspoon of white pepper

Directions

- Boil potatoes, let simmer until tender in 20 minutes.
- Add the snap peas in the same water during the last minute.
- Drain. Rinse under cold water.
- Boil the eggs.
- Stir in olive oil, champagne vinegar, mustard, shallot, dill, salt, sugar, white pepper, and horseradish, tasting and adjust.
- Serve and enjoy with the vegetables salad.

Roasted black bean burgers

The roasted black bean burger features variety of fruits and vegetables typically mango, avocado, tabasco, tomatoes among others, making a perfect Mediterranean Sea diet.

Ingredients

- 1 ripe avocado
- 1½ red onions
- 200g of mixed mushrooms
- Chipotle tabasco sauce
- 4 tablespoons of natural yoghurt
- 100g of rye bread
- Ground coriander
- 1 x 400 g tin of black beans
- 4 sprigs of fresh coriander
- Olive oil
- 40g of mature cheddar cheese
- 1 ripe mango
- 4 soft rolls
- 100g of ripe cherry tomatoes
- 1 lime

Directions

- Preheat the oven ready to 400°F.
- Place 1 onion in a food processor with rye bread mushrooms, and ground coriander process until fine.
- Drain, pulse in the black beans
- Season lightly with sea salt and black pepper.
- Divide into 4 and shape into patties.
- Rub with oil and dust with ground coriander.
- Transfer to oiled baking tray let roast for 25 minutes, until dark and crispy.
- Top with the Cheddar, then warm the rolls.
- Combine the onions and tomatoes in a bowl.
- Squeeze over the lime juice with a bit of Tabasco.
- Season to taste.
- Halve the warm rolls and divide the yoghurt between the bases, and half of the salsa, avocado, mango, and coriander leaves.
- Top with the burgers and the balance of salsa and press down lightly.
- Serve and enjoy.

Brilliant bhaji burger

Ingredients

- 2 fresh green chilies
- 75g of paneer cheese
- 200g of butternut squash
- Mango chutney
- 4cm piece of ginger
- 100g of plain flour
- 1 lime
- 2 teaspoons of Rogan josh curry paste
- 2 cloves of garlic
- 2 uncooked poppadum
- Olive oil
- 4 soft burger buns
- 1 red onion
- 1 big bunch of fresh coriander
- 75g of natural yoghurt
- 1 baby gem lettuce

Directions

- Combine onion, garlic, chilies, and coriander stalks in a bowl.

- Add paneer with squash, ginger.
- Sprinkle in the flour and a pinch of sea salt and black pepper.
- Squeeze over the lime juice.
- Add the curry paste and water, mix.
- Drizzle 2 tablespoons of oil into a large non-stick frying pan over a medium heat.
- Divide the mixture into 4 portions and place in the pan.
- Let fry for 16 minutes, turning every few minutes.
- Then pound most of the coriander leaves to a paste in a pestle, muddle in the yoghurt, season.
- Divide the coriander yoghurt between the bases and inside bun-lids, then break up the poppadoms and sprinkle over.
- Place a crispy bhaji burger on top of each bun-base.
- Add a dollop of mango chutney, coriander leaves, and the lettuce.
- Serve and enjoy chilled.

Summer Tagliatelle

Ingredients

- 1 potato
- ½ a clove of garlic
- 200g of delicate summer vegetables
- 50g of blanched almonds
- 300g of Tagliatelle
- Extra virgin olive oil
- 25g of Parmesan cheese
- ¼ of a lemon
- 1 bunch of fresh basil
- 125g of green beans

Directions

- Place most of the basil leaves into a pestle pulse to a paste with a pinch of sea salt.
- Add in the garlic with pounded almonds until fine.
- Muddle in 4 tablespoons of oil with parmesan, squeeze of lemon juice.
- Season accordingly.

- Place sliced potatoes and beans in a pan of boiling salted water with Tagliatelle.
- Let cook as per the pasta packet Directions.
- Add delicate summer vegetables to the pan for the last 3 minutes.
- Drain, and keep some cooking water, then toss with the pesto, loosening with a splash of reserved water.
- Drizzle with 1 tablespoon of oil, complete with basil.
- Serve and enjoy with crunchy salad.

Roasted tomato risotto

Ingredients

- 450g of Arborio risotto rice
- 80g of Parmesan cheese
- 1 bulb of fennel
- 1 bulb of garlic
- ½ a bunch of fresh thyme
- 150ml of dry white vermouth
- Olive oil
- 1.2 liters of organic vegetable stock
- 1 onion
- 2 knobs of unsalted butter
- 6 large ripe tomatoes

Directions

- Preheat the oven ready to 350°F.
- Remove tomatoes seeds, place in a snug-fitting baking dish with cut sides up with garlic bulb.
- Spread with thyme sprigs.
- Drizzle with 1 tablespoon of oil.
- Season with sea salt, let roast until starting to burst open.

- Bring the stock to a simmer.
- Place onions with olive oil and knob of butter in a large pan on a medium heat. butter.
- Cook until softened, stirring occasionally.
- Stir in the rice, toast for 2 minutes.
- Pour in the vermouth, stir until absorbed.
- Add the stock let it be fully absorbed, then add another, stirring constantly until the rice is cooked in 18 minutes.
- Beat in the remaining knob of butter, Parmesan.
- Season and turn off the heat.
- Let rest for 2 minutes.
- Divide the risotto between warm plates, place a tomato in the center with sweet garlic and the herby fennel.
- Serve and enjoy.

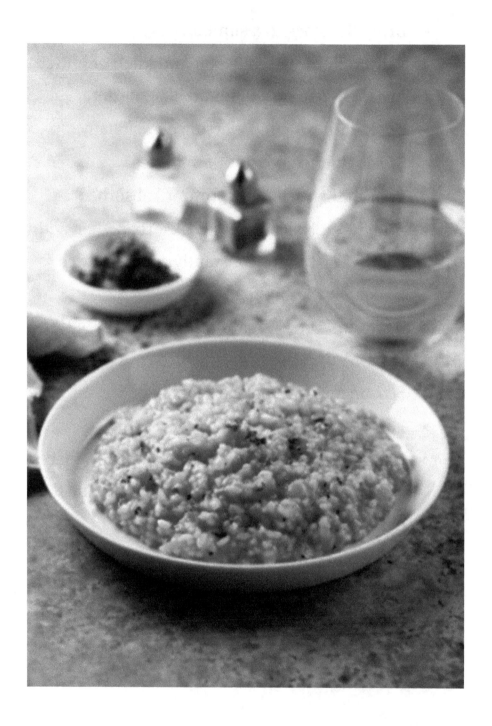

Veggie pad Thai

Ingredients

- 320g of crunchy vegetables
- Sesame oil
- Olive oil
- 80g of silken tofu
- Low-salt soy sauce
- 150g of rice noodles
- ½ a mixed bunch of fresh basil, mint and coriander
- 2 teaspoons of tamarind paste
- 2 cloves of garlic
- ½ a cos lettuce
- 2 teaspoons of sweet chili sauce
- 2 limes
- 20g of unsalted peanuts
- 1 shallot
- 80g of beansprouts
- 2 large free-range eggs
- Dried chili flakes

Directions

- Start by cook the noodles according to the packet Directions.

- Drain any excess water, toss with 1 teaspoon of sesame oil.

- Toast the peanuts in a large non-stick frying pan on a medium heat until golden.

- Blend in a pestle until fine, place into a bowl.

- Bash the garlic to a paste with the tofu.

- Add sesame oil with soy, tamarind paste, and chili sauce.

- Muddle in half the lime juice.

- Place slices of shallot in a frying pan over a high heat.

- Dry-fry the crunchy veggies for 4 minutes.

- Add the noodles together with sauce, beansprouts, and splash of water, toss over heat for 1 minute.

- Wipe out the pan, crack in the eggs let cook in a little olive oil, sprinkled with a pinch of chili flakes.

- Place lettuce in the bowls with eggs on top and pick over the herbs.
- Serve and enjoy with lime wedges.

Pea and ricotta stuffed courgettes

Ingredients

- 2 cloves of garlic
- 4 sprigs of fresh mint
- olive oil
- 100g of ricotta cheese
- 50g of mature Cheddar cheese
- 300g of basmati rice
- 1 lemon
- 8 baby courgettes, with flowers
- 400g of ripe cherry tomatoes
- red wine vinegar
- 150g of fresh or frozen peas
- 4 spring onions
- 8 black olives
- 1 fresh red chili

Directions

- Preheat the oven ready to 400°F.
- Process the mint leaves in a food processor with peas, ricotta, and Cheddar.

- Squeeze in the lemon juice with black pepper, blend until smooth.
- Taste and adjust the seasoning.
- Fill each courgette flower with the mixture, seal the petals.
- Place the tomatoes, onions, and olives roasting tray.
- Drizzle with 2 tablespoons each of oil and vinegar, season with pepper.
- Stir in the rice and boiling water, bring to the boil, stirring occasionally.
- Bake the courgettes inside rice for 20 minutes until golden.
- Serve and enjoy with summery salad

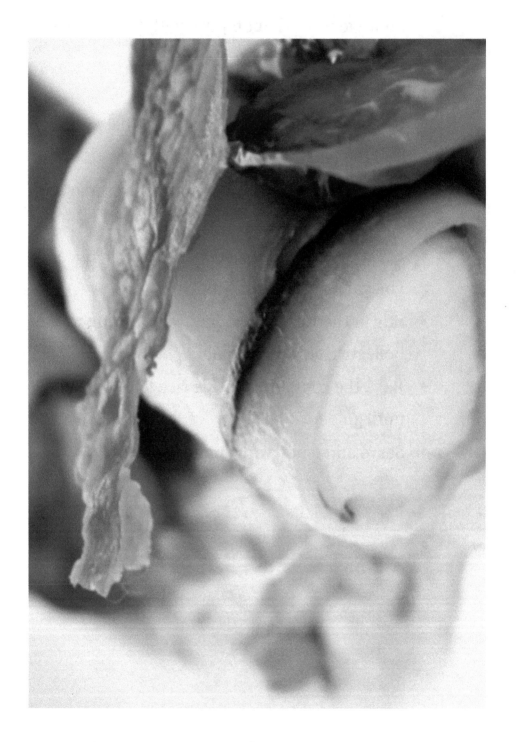

Veggie pasties

Ingredients

- 1 large free-range egg
- 250g of unsalted butter
- 200g of swede
- 1 pinch of dried rosemary
- 400g of potatoes
- 500g of strong flour
- 1 onion
- 500g of mixed mushrooms

Directions

- Tear the mushrooms into a bowl, scatter over 15g of sea salt, leave for 30 minutes, scrunching occasionally.
- Place flour with a pinch of salt into a bowl.
- Rub in the butter.
- Make a well in the middle, pour in cold water, mix, pat dry.
- Wrap in Clingfilm and refrigerate for 1 hour.
- Squeeze to salty liquid after 30 minutes.

- Mix the veggies with the mushrooms, rosemary and pinches of black pepper.
- Preheat the oven to 350°F.
- Divide the pastry into 8, then roll out into rounds.
- Divide up the filling, then scrunch and pile it to one side of the middle.
- Brush the exposed pastry with beaten egg, fold over and press the edges down, seal with your thumb. Egg wash.
- Place on a lined baking sheet let bake for 40 minutes.
- Serve and enjoy with watercress.

Asparagus quiche and soup

Ingredients

- 1.5 liters of organic vegetable stock
- 125g of whole meal flour
- 2 onions
- 150g of mature Cheddar cheese
- 125g of unsalted butter
- 7 large free-range eggs
- 1kg of asparagus
- 150g of ricotta cheese
- Olive oil
- 125g of plain flour
- 2 large potatoes
- ½ a bunch of fresh thyme

Directions

- Preheat the oven to 350°F.
- Put flours into a bowl with pinch of sea salt, rub in the butter.
- Make a well in the middle, crack in one of the eggs, mix with cold water, pat dry and bring together.

- Place between two large sheets of greaseproof paper, flatten, chill for 30 minutes.
- Roll out the pastry between the sheets, line a loose-bottomed tart tin with the pastry, bake for 20 minutes.
- Place asparagus and oil in a large pan over a medium heat.
- Add the potatoes with onions, thyme leaves cook until lightly golden, stirring regularly.
- Pour in the stock, boil, then simmer for 15 minutes.
- Blend until smooth, sieve.
- Season to taste with salt and black pepper.
- Beat the remaining eggs in a bowl with a pinch of salt and pepper.
- Add the ricotta with Cheddar and remaining thyme leaves.
- Stir the asparagus into the egg mixture and tip into the tart case.
- Let bake for 40 minutes.
- Serve and enjoy.

Summer vegetable blanket pie

Ingredients

- 320g of ripe cherry tomatoes
- 4 cloves of garlic
- 1 tablespoon of fennel seeds
- Olive oil
- 1 pinch of saffron
- 320g of potatoes
- 320g of butternut squash
- 320g of courgettes
- 1 tablespoon of sesame seeds
- ½ x 700g jar of chickpeas
- 1 large leek
- Extra virgin olive oil
- 8 sheets of filo pastry
- 1 preserved lemon
- 1 tablespoon of red wine vinegar
- 400g of natural yoghurt
- 1 teaspoon of rose harissa
- 50g of dried sour cherries

Directions

- Sieve the yogurt through into a bowl, then leave to drain.

- Season the tomatoes with sea salt and black pepper.

- Drizzle with extra virgin olive oil and the vinegar, then toss, let macerate.

- Preheat the oven to 375°F.

- Place garlic slices in a large frying pan on a medium heat with the fennel seeds and olive oil.

- Fry briefly, stirring regularly.

- Add potatoes, leek, and courgette let cook covered for 15 minutes.

- Add the chickpeas, season with a pinch of salt and pepper.

- Add lemon to the pan with a drizzle of juice from the jar, and the harissa.

- Continue to fry for 15 more minutes, stirring occasionally.

- Cover the sour cherries and saffron with boiling water, add tomatoes, reserving the macerating juices.
- Lay the filo out flat, then brush with tomato juices.
- Scatter over the sesame seeds and bake for 25 minutes
- Serve and enjoy with the pie.

Allotment cottage pie

The delicious taste of the allotment cottage pie will surprise anyone's taste buds. It is fully packed with variety of nutrients and a perfect Mediterranean Sea diet choice.

Ingredients

- 1 teaspoon of Marmite
- 2 large leeks
- 3 carrots
- 1 x 400g tin of green lentils
- 1 splash of semi-skimmed milk
- 10g of dried porcini mushrooms
- 500g of swede
- 500g of celeriac
- Olive oil
- 3 sprigs of fresh rosemary
- 1 onion
- 3 tablespoons of tomato purée
- 1 teaspoon cumin seeds
- 2kg of potatoes
- 40g of unsalted butter

Directions

- In a blender, cover the porcini with hot water.
- Drizzle oil into a large casserole pan over a medium heat.
- Fry the rosemary for 1 minute to crisp up.
- Add the cumin seeds together with prepared veggies to flavored oil.
- Season with sea salt and black pepper, cook for 30 minutes, stirring regularly.
- Cook the potatoes in a pan of boiling salted water until tender.
- Drain and mash with butter and milk, then season.
- Preheat the oven to 375°F.
- Add onions, marmite, tomato puree, blend until smooth.
- Pour into the veggie pan and cook for 20 minutes, stirring regularly.
- Place the lentils into the veg pan, boil, season to taste.
- Spoon over the mash, place on a tray.

- Let bake for 30 minutes, or until bubbling at the edges.
- Sprinkle over the crispy rosemary.
- Serve and enjoy with seasonal greens.

Sticky onion tart

The stick onion tart is quite flavorful with garlic and the onion itself. Above and beyond, this recipe is easy to make.

Ingredients

- 4 tablespoons of cider vinegar
- 4 medium onions
- 320g of sheet of all-butter puff pastry
- 50g of unsalted butter
- 8 cloves of garlic
- 4 sprigs of fresh thyme
- 4 fresh bay leaves
- 2 tablespoons of soft dark brown sugar

Directions

- Preheat the oven ready to 425°F.
- Place butter in an ovenproof frying pan on a medium heat.
- Add thyme leaves with the bay, sugar, vinegar, and water.
- Place the onion halves in the pan, cut side down with garlic in between.
- Season with sea salt and black pepper.

- Cover, over low heat and steam for 10 minutes to soften the onions, uncover cook until liquid starts to caramelize.
- Place the pastry over the onions, placed to the edge of the pan.
- Let bake for 35 minutes, until golden brown.
- Serve and enjoy.

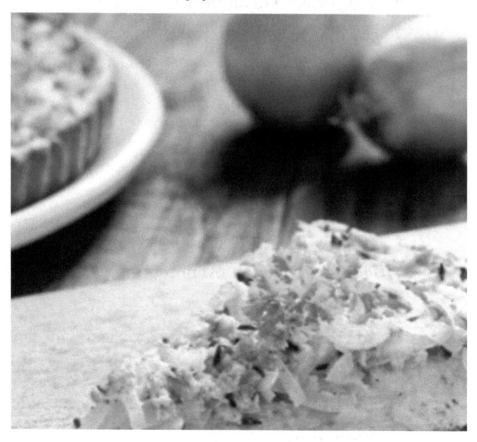

Tomato curry

Ingredients

- 2 teaspoons of mango chutney
- 1 onion
- 1.2kg of ripe mixed tomatoes
- 1 pinch of saffron
- 1 teaspoon of mustard seeds
- 1 teaspoon of fenugreek seeds
- 1 x 400g tin of light coconut milk
- 20g of flaked almonds
- 4 cloves of garlic
- 1 teaspoon of cumin seeds
- 4cm piece of ginger
- 2 fresh red chilies
- Olive oil
- 1 handful of fresh curry leaves

Directions

- Prick the tomatoes, plunge into fast-boiling water briefly.
- Peel the skin.

- Cover the saffron with boiling water and leave to infuse.
- Toast the almonds in a large non-stick frying pan over a medium heat until golden.
- Transfer to a small bowl and place the pan back on the heat.
- Drizzle 1 tablespoon of oil into the pan, add curry leaves with all the spices.
- Add onions with garlic, ginger, and chili to the pan, let fry for 3 minutes, stirring constantly.
- Add the tomatoes with the coconut milk and saffron water, let simmer for 20 minutes covered.
- Add mango chutney halfway.
- Season to taste with sea salt and black pepper, scatter over the almonds.
- Serve and enjoy with fluffy rice.

Vegetable chili

Ingredients

- 2 sweet potatoes
- 1 x 400g tin of cannellini beans
- 3 mixed-color peppers
- 4 large ripe tomatoes
- 1 lemon
- 1 bunch of fresh mint
- 4 tablespoons of natural yoghurt
- Olive oil
- 1 teaspoon of cumin seeds
- 1 teaspoon of smoked paprika
- 2 red onions
- 4 small flour tortillas
- 4 cloves of garlic
- Hot chili sauce
- 250g of black rice

Directions

- Preheat a griddle pan ready to high temperature.

- Drizzle 1 tablespoon of oil into a large casserole pan over a medium-low heat.
- Stir in the cumin with paprika, garlic, lemon zest, and grilled vegetables, stirring regularly.
- Add the beans and water, add chili sauce.
- Season with sea salt and black pepper let simmer for 30 minutes.
- Cook the rice in a pan of boiling salted water according to the packet Directions.
- Pick 2 sprigs of mint leaves and chop with the salsa veggie, toss with the lemon juice.
- Season to taste with salt and pepper.
- Warm the tortillas on the griddle and ripple shakes of chili sauce through the yoghurt.
- Serve and enjoy with black rice.

Chicken and vegetable stir-fry

Ingredients

- 2 carrots
- ½ of a red onion
- 1 red pepper
- 80g of purple sprouting broccoli
- 1 tablespoon of reduced-salt soy sauce
- 80g of mixed mushrooms
- 1 free-range chicken breast
- 1 teaspoon of sesame seeds
- 1 tablespoon of sesame oil
- 4cm of piece of ginger
- 1 teaspoon of Chinese five-spice
- 1 teaspoon of vegetable oil
- Sprigs of fresh coriander
- 1 fresh red chili
- 1 clove of garlic
- 130g of baby corn
- 80g of mange tout
- 2 whole wheat noodle nests
- 1 tablespoon of black bean sauce

Directions

- Place the chicken into a bowl with the Chinese five-spice and sesame oil, toss.
- Place a large non-stick frying pan over a medium-high heat with the vegetable oil.
- Add the garlic together with the ginger and chili, toss briefly.
- Add the chicken let stir-fry for 2 minutes until golden.
- Add all the vegetables, let stir-fry for more 4 minutes.
- Cook the noodles as instructed on the package in a large pan of boiling salted water.
- Transfer the noodles to the pan, add soy with black bean sauce, toss to coat.
- Scatter over the sesame seeds and coriander.
- Serve and enjoy.

Roasted vegetable roots

Much as there are various ways one can roast veggies, the Mediterranean style is mega for a delicious and aromatic flavor with garlic taking the lead.

Ingredients

- 12 parsnips
- 3kg of potatoes
- 16 carrots
- ½ a bunch of fresh rosemary
- 1 bulb of garlic

Directions

- Begin by preheat your oven ready to 375°F.
- Cook potatoes with parsnips and carrots in a large pan of boiling salted water for 8 minutes.
- Drain any excess water in a colander let steam dry.
- Remove the carrots and parsnips put to one side, shakes the colander.
- Add 4 tablespoons of olive oil to two large roasting trays.
- Season each with sea salt and black pepper.

- Squash the garlic bulb, divide between the trays with the rosemary sprigs.
- Place in the veggies, red wine vinegar, toss to coat.
- Let roast for 40 minutes.
- Remove and squash with a fish slice to burst the skins.
- Place back in the oven for 20 minutes.
- Serve and enjoy.

Beetroot curry

What a blessing to add onto your body blood. Beet root is a gift to replenish blood in the body; as such, this recipe cannot be underestimated among Mediterranean Sea diets with earthly flavors.

Ingredients

- 1 teaspoon of hot curry powder
- 3 cloves of garlic
- 2 tablespoons of desiccated coconut
- 3 cloves of garlic
- 5cm of piece of ginger
- vegetable oil
- 2 teaspoons of black mustard seeds
- 1 kg mixed beets
- 250g of ripe cherry tomatoes
- 7g of dried curry leaves
- ½ a bunch of fresh coriander
- 320g of wild rice
- 6 spring onions
- 14g of dried curry leaves
- 5cm of piece of ginger

- 1 x 400ml tin of light coconut milk
- 1 lemon
- 1 lime
- 2 fresh long red chilies

Directions

- Place a large pan over a medium heat.
- Add the curry leaves with the curry powder, mustard seeds, and coconut, let toast for 2 minute. Transfer to a food processor and blend well.
- Add spring onions to the food processor with garlic, ginger, and vegetable oil.
- Pulse to forms a paste.
- Place the pan back on the hob over a medium heat.
- Add the paste cook briefly, add beetroot.
- Lower heat and cook until sticky and gnarly, stirring often.
- Add the cherry tomatoes and cook for 5 minutes, then break them with the back of a spoon.
- Cook the rice as instructed on the packet.

- Stir in the coconut milk with a squeeze of lemon juice.
- Raise the heat let cook for 5 minutes.
- Season to taste.
- Place a frying pan over a medium heat with oil.
- Add all the temper ingredients let heat for 2 minutes.
- Turn off the heat, transfer into a bowl lined with kitchen paper.
- Serve the curry with the rice and temper and or coriander leaves scattered on top.
- Serve and enjoy.

Brick lane burger

Everyone likes to enjoy a delicious burger, isn't it? If yes, then this Mediterranean Sea diet recipe is a must try for you. It has great flavors derived from onions, garlic and ginger.

Ingredients

- 200g of butternut squash
- 2 cloves of garlic
- 2 fresh green chilies
- 100g of paneer cheese
- Mango chutney
- 1 big bunch of fresh coriander
- 150g of gram flour
- 6 burger buns
- 2 teaspoons of ground turmeric
- 3 poppadoms
- 2 baby gem lettuce
- 1 carrot
- 2 teaspoons of ground cumin
- 2 red onions
- 2 limes

- Olive oil
- 100ml of natural yoghurt
- 5cm of piece of ginger
- 1 fresh red chili

Directions

- Preheat the oven to 350°F.
- Place onions, carrots, paneer, garlic, ginger, and coriander into a large mixing bowl.
- Place flour together with the turmeric and cumin.
- Season with sea salt and black pepper, squeeze in the juice of 1 lime with water, mix with your hands.
- Divide into 6, then shape and squash into patties.
- Drizzle with bit of oil into a large non-stick frying pan over a medium heat.
- Let fry the patties for 3 minutes on each side or until golden.
- Remove to a baking tray for 10 minutes or until cooked.

- Pestle the remaining coriander leaves, setting aside a handful.
- Add a pinch of salt, then bash to a paste. Squeeze in the juice of lime, stir in the yoghurt.
- Spoon a little coriander yoghurt over the base and inside lid of each burger bun.
- Crumble the poppadoms, sprinkle over the yoghurt, then sit a patty on top of each base and spread with 1 tablespoon of mango chutney.
- Top with a handful of lettuce and the reserved coriander leaves.
- Sprinkle with red chili
- Serve and enjoy.

Summer vegetable lasagna

Ingredients

- Olive oil
- ½ x 30g tin of anchovies in oil
- 6 cloves of garlic
- 500g of fresh lasagne sheets
- 700g of asparagus
- 1 lemon
- Sprigs of fresh thyme
- 500g of frozen peas
- 300g of frozen broad beans
- Parmesan cheese
- 1 bunch of spring onions
- 1 big bunch of fresh mint
- 300ml of single cream
- 300m of organic vegetable stock
- 2 x 250g tubs of cottage cheese

Directions

- Preheat the grill to full temperature.
- Pour oil from the anchovy tin into a large frying pan over a high heat

- Add the spring onions and anchovies.
- Add crushed garlic, toss well.
- Add asparagus stems to the pan, keep tips for later.
- Season with sea salt and black pepper.
- Add a splash of boiling water, let cook for a few minutes, stirring occasionally.
- Add the peas together with the broad beans, mint, lemon zest, and the cream to the pan.
- Squash, then season with salt and pepper.
- Pour in the stock and bring to the boil.
- Stir in 1 tub of cottage cheese.
- Place a roasting tray over a medium heat.
- Cover the bottom of the tray with the vegetable mixture, then top with a layer of lasagna sheets, and Parmesan grating.
- Repeat the layers with the rest of the vegetable mixture and pasta, use lasagne sheets to finish.
- Mix the remaining tub of cottage cheese with splash of water.

- Toss the reserved asparagus with a drizzle of oil.
- Strip over the thyme leaves.
- Turn the heat under the tray up to high and cook until the lasagne starts to bubble, place under the grill on the middle shelf for 8 minutes.
- Serve and enjoy.

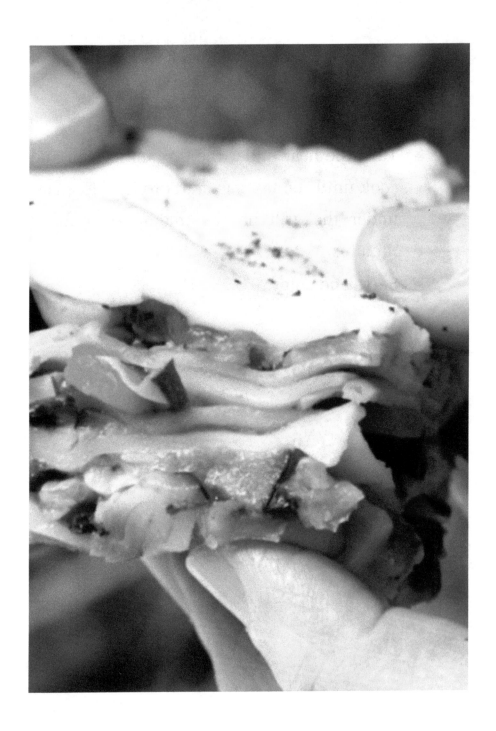

CPSIA information can be obtained
at www.ICGtesting.com
Printed in the USA
BVHW091048090621
609091BV00008B/691